Children's Fun Activity & Coloring Book

BY RICHARD SCHMIDT

Copyright

Children's Fun Activity & Coloring Book

Cover design by Richard Schmidt / Plaque Pixie Books
Book design by Richard Schmidt

Printed in the United States of America

First Printing: July 2013

Plaque Pixie Books LTD.

Children's Fun Activity & Coloring Book

BY RICHARD SCHMIDT

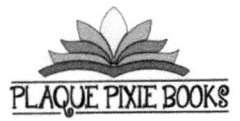

PLAQUE PIXIE BOOKS

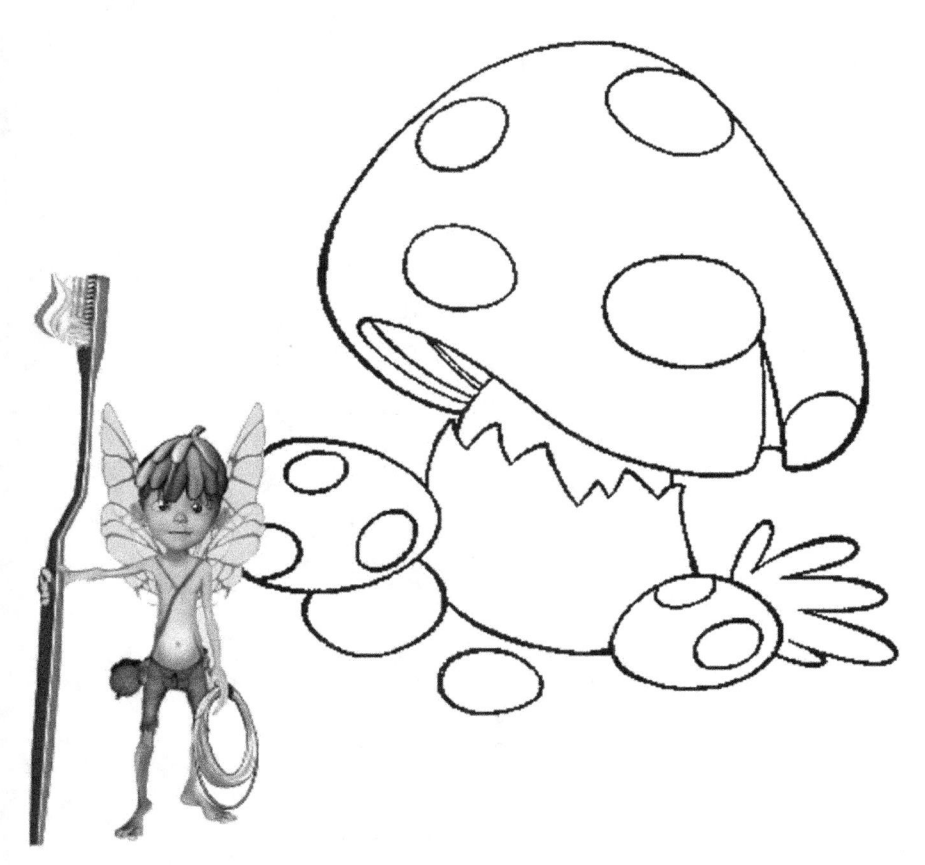

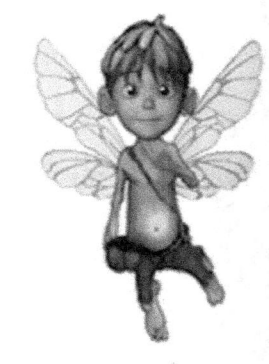

```
T N E M T N I O P P A F G E B
A S S I S T A N T C B L N R I
E Y A R X Y A P S A R O I U T
C N A E L C N Y M V U S L T E
I E B R A C E S U I S S L N N
F E L J A T L S G T H V I E I
F D A E A L N T N Y C L F D N
O L R S I W C E T I C A T B A
R E O R F E M N M E R C F I C
O M D U J U E I R T A O P B P
S A M N R V N M I R A L O M O
I N I T E I W A T E R E C Q L
C E S R A N D X T N W O R C I
N N P P H T E E T L I G H T S
I N S U R A N C E N E I G Y H
```

APPOINTMENT	EXTRACT	NEEDLE
ASSISTANT	FILLING	NURSE
BIB	FLOSS	OFFICE
BITE	FLOURIDE	ORAL
BRACES	GUMS	PAIN
BRUSH	HYGIENE	PAY
CANINE	INCISOR	POLISH
CAVITY	INJECT	PREVENT
CLEAN	INSTRUMENTS	RECLINE
CROWN	INSURANCE	RINSE
DENTURE	JAW	TEETH
DRILL	LIGHT	TREATMENT
ENAMEL	LOCAL	WATER
EXAMINE	MOLAR	XRAY

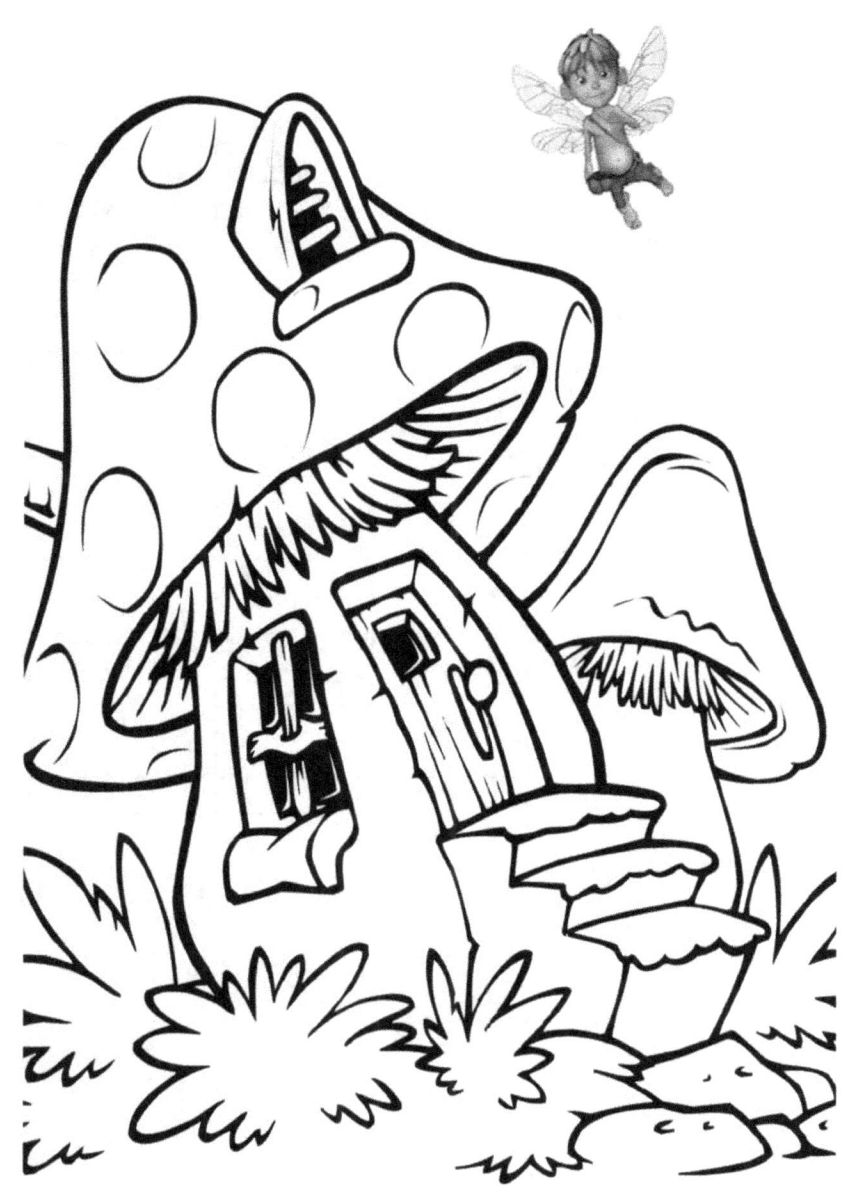

DENTAL CARE
Crossword

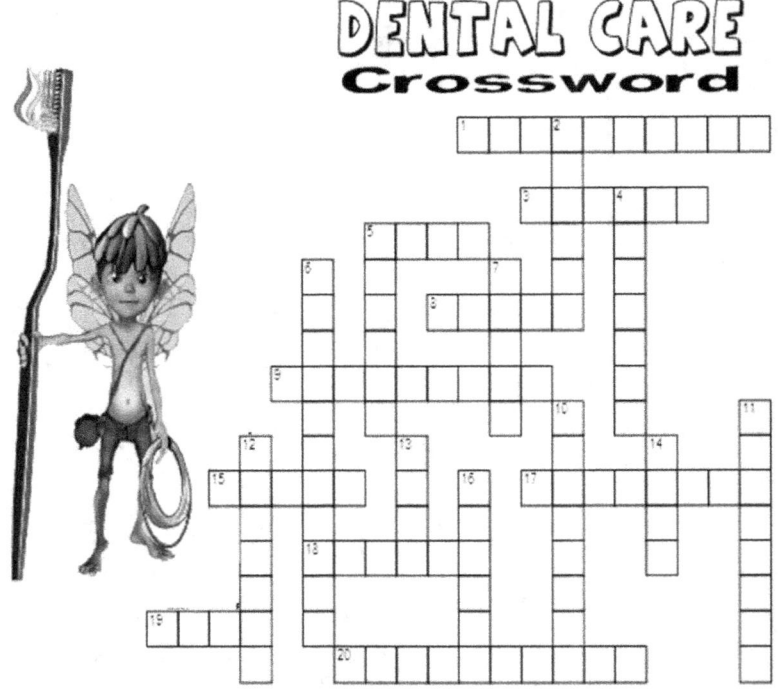

ACROSS

1. A common tool people use to clean their teeth
3. They straighten your smile
5. To bite and grind with the teeth
8. The kind of tooth found at the back of the mouth
9. A liquid to rinse the mouth that freshens breath
15. More than one tooth
17. A chemical that helps to prevent cavities
18. The outside part of a tooth
19. Pink tissue surrounding the teeth
20. Cleanser for teeth

DOWN

2. A crusty build-up on teeth
4. A meeting with your dentist to see if you need any work done
5. A hole in a tooth
6. An arranged day and time to meet with someone
7. String used to clean between teeth
10. Dentists add these to fix teeth that have holes
11. Making less-dirty
12. Tooth Doctor
13. A test
14. Used to take a picture of the inside of someone's teeth
16. Makes things look glossy

Dental Word Search

Can you find all the hidden words? They can be up, down or diagonal.

WORDS:

TEACH
HANDS
MATH
FEEL
HARD
STRAIGHTEN
PATIENTS
TOOTH
SCHOOL

CHILDREN
SCIENCE
LIFETIME
LOOK
WATCH
FIX
LONG
CONTACT
VISIT

```
F  G  I  P  T  Z  C  D  E  H
W  X  J  K  E  H  A  N  D  S
S  I  T  T  A  V  Q  U  V  C
T  H  C  S  C  H  O  O  L  I
R  M  A  T  H  T  I  D  R  E
A  Y  H  R  N  F  E  E  L  N
I  P  B  O  D  Y  A  M  O  C
G  L  W  A  T  C  H  Z  O  E
H  O  O  D  G  J  K  M  K  N
T  N  C  O  N  T  A  C  T  X
E  G  G  H  K  F  I  X  I  P
N  G  L  I  F  E  T  I  M  E
A  C  P  A  T  I  E  N  T  S
O  N  H  Q  R  O  U  V  N  O
A  D  B  I  S  P  O  E  N  Z
E  N  O  D  L  S  H  T  O  L
E  N  C  P  E  D  F  E  H  M
V  I  S  I  T  Y  R  B  O  Z
T  I  E  N  T  P  A  E  N  Q
K  N  O  G  F  A  P  Z  N  P
```

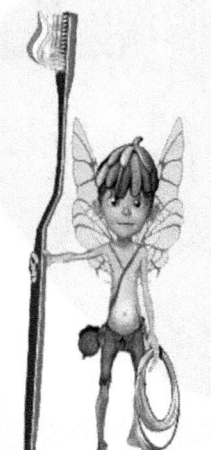

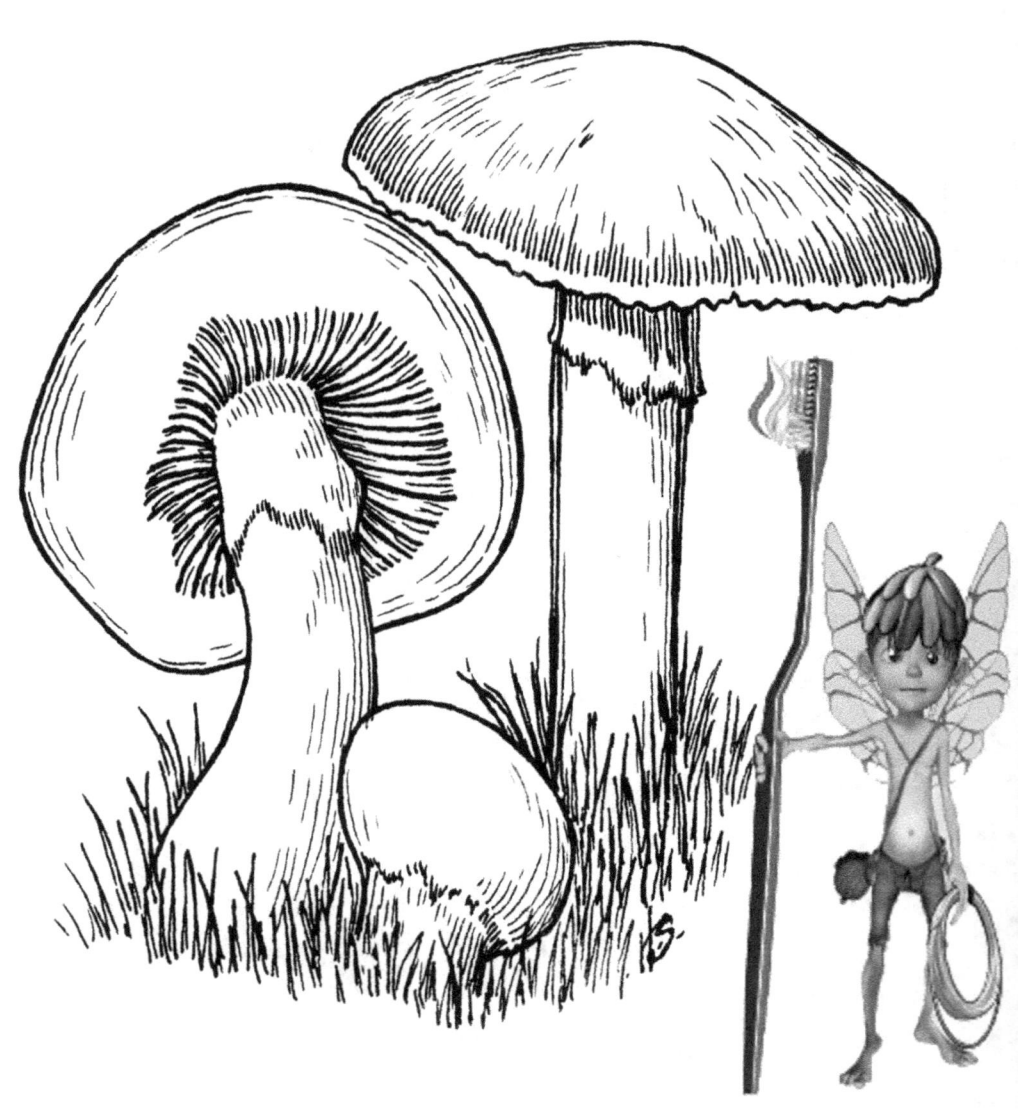

```
F E C B R A C E S O C S P I K
S S R A L O M O L G A E D L J
M N L L I R D M N S V R L L H
I E M W P N S I S V I U Y E W
L E O X B E L D W U T T D M I
E D U D I L Z E I V Y N I A S
Z L T V I L E W S P N E P N D
M E H F P O F E H L S D S E O
Q B W F N W V L D S R U U M M
W W A N V S O H U I O H C I T
A G S N I A C O V O N I I R I
T L H C R O W N S P R G B R P
E B R U S H E D S T A I N O S
R T O N G U E H T E E T D R A
J R U G N I N E T H G I T E O
```

BICUSPID   NEEDLE
BLEEDING   NOVOCAIN
BRACES   SMILE
BRUSH   SPIT
CAVITY   STAIN
CROWNS   SWISH
CUSPIDS   SWOLLEN
DENTURES   TEETH
DRILL   TIGHTENING
ENAMEL   TONGUE
FILLING   WATER
FLUORIDE   WISDOM
MIRROR
MOLARS
MOUTHWASH

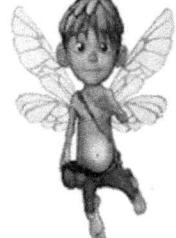

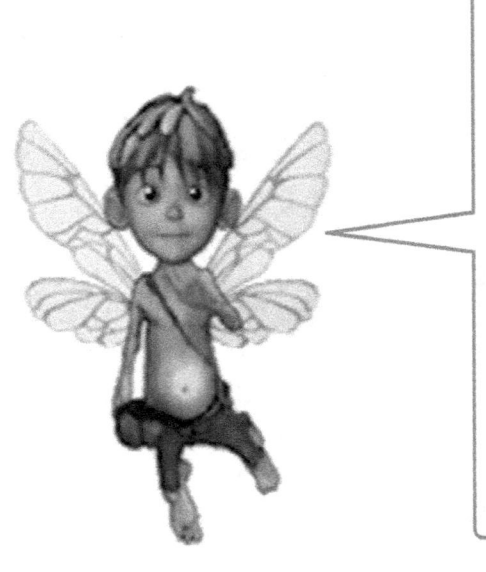

USE THE CHART
BELOW TO KEEP
TRACK OF
YOUR DAILY
BRUSHING

The Plaque Pixie BRUSH CHART

	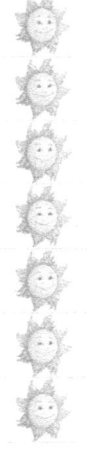	
MONDAY		
TUESDAY		
WEDNESDAY		
THURSDAY		
FRIDAY		
SATURDAY		
SUNDAY		

the Plaque Pixie's
Dental Health Challenge

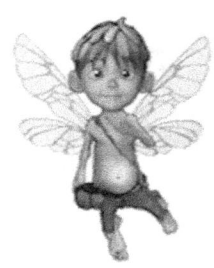

1. Soft, strong thread used to clean between the teeth
   A. Floss B. Cavity C. Dentist D. Root

2. A soft, sticky, whitish film attached to tooth surfaces
   A. Enamel B. Molars C. Plaque D. Gums

3. A brush for cleaning the teeth
   A. Cavity B. Enamel C. Toothbrush D. Molars

4. A hole in the tooth caused by tooth decay
   A. Cavity B. Root C. Gums D. Molars

5. A person whose profession is dentistry
   A. Cavity B. Dentist C. Floss D. Toothbrush

6. A paste for cleaning teeth
   A. Toothpaste B. Enamel C. Dentist D. Gums

7. The part of the tooth below the gums
   A. Toothbrush B. Gums C. Enamel D. Root

8. The hardest substance in your body
   A. Molars B. Cavity C. Plaque D. Enamel

9. Large back teeth used for grinding your food
   A. Gums B. Molars C. Enamel D. Toothbrush

10. The pink tissue at the bottom of teeth
    A. Toothpaste B. Floss C. Cavity D. Gums

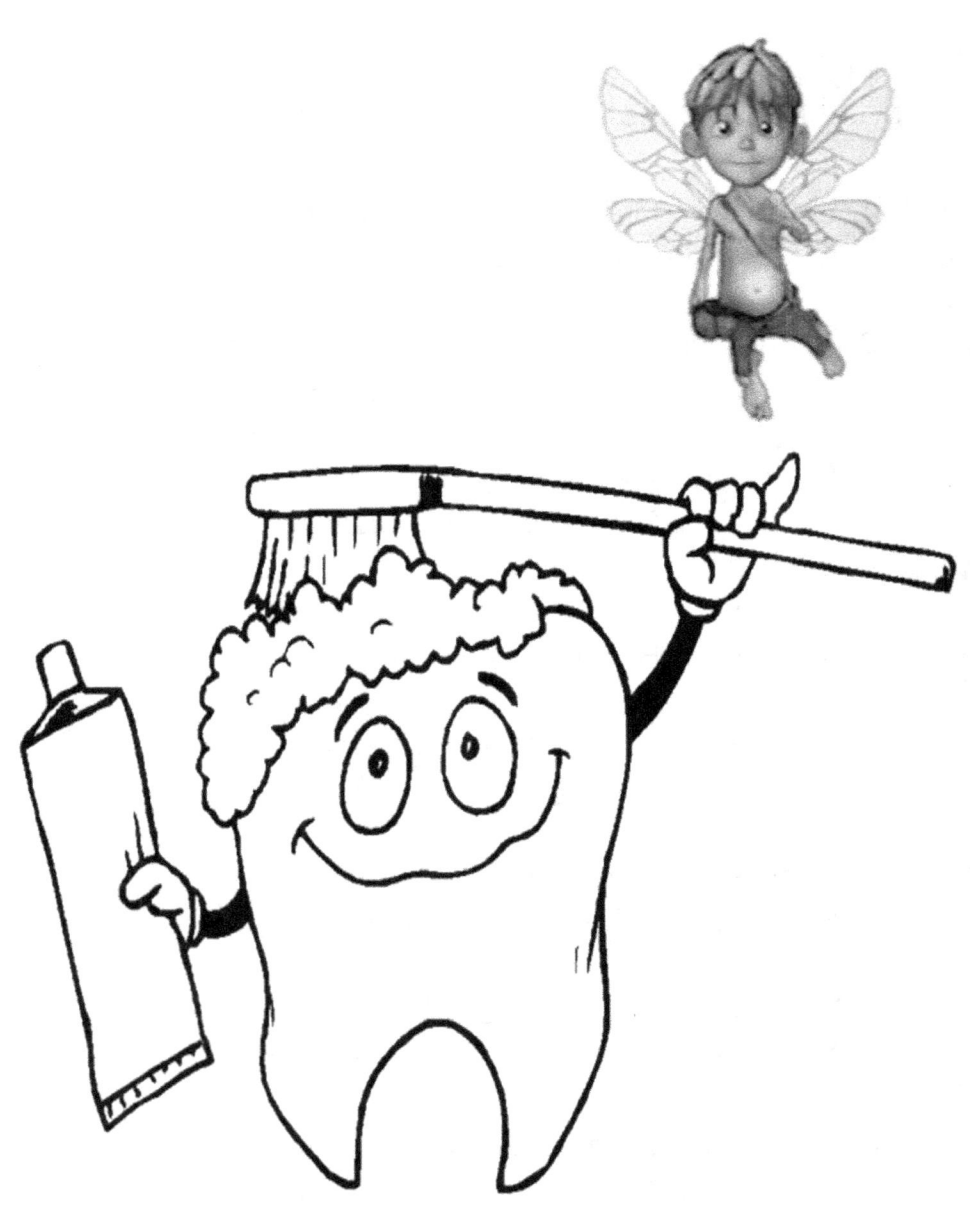

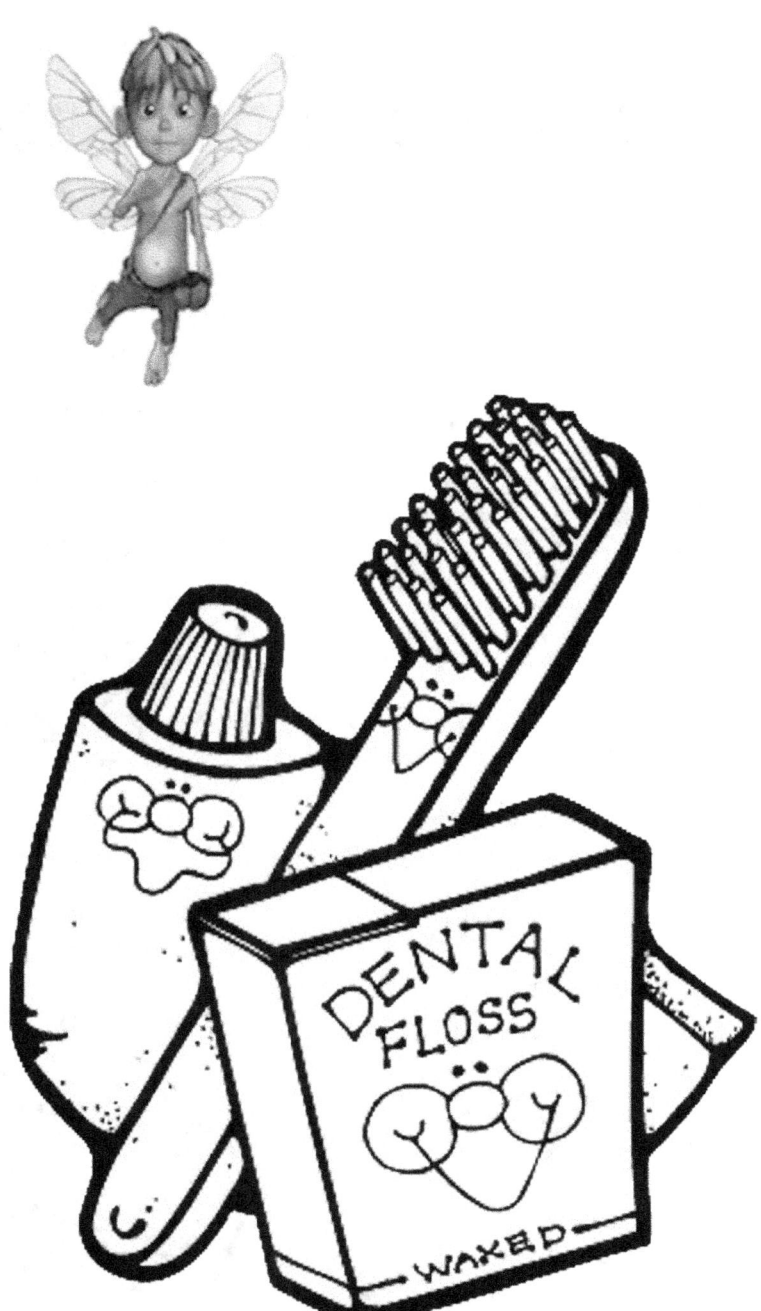

WHICH ONE IS DIFFERENT?

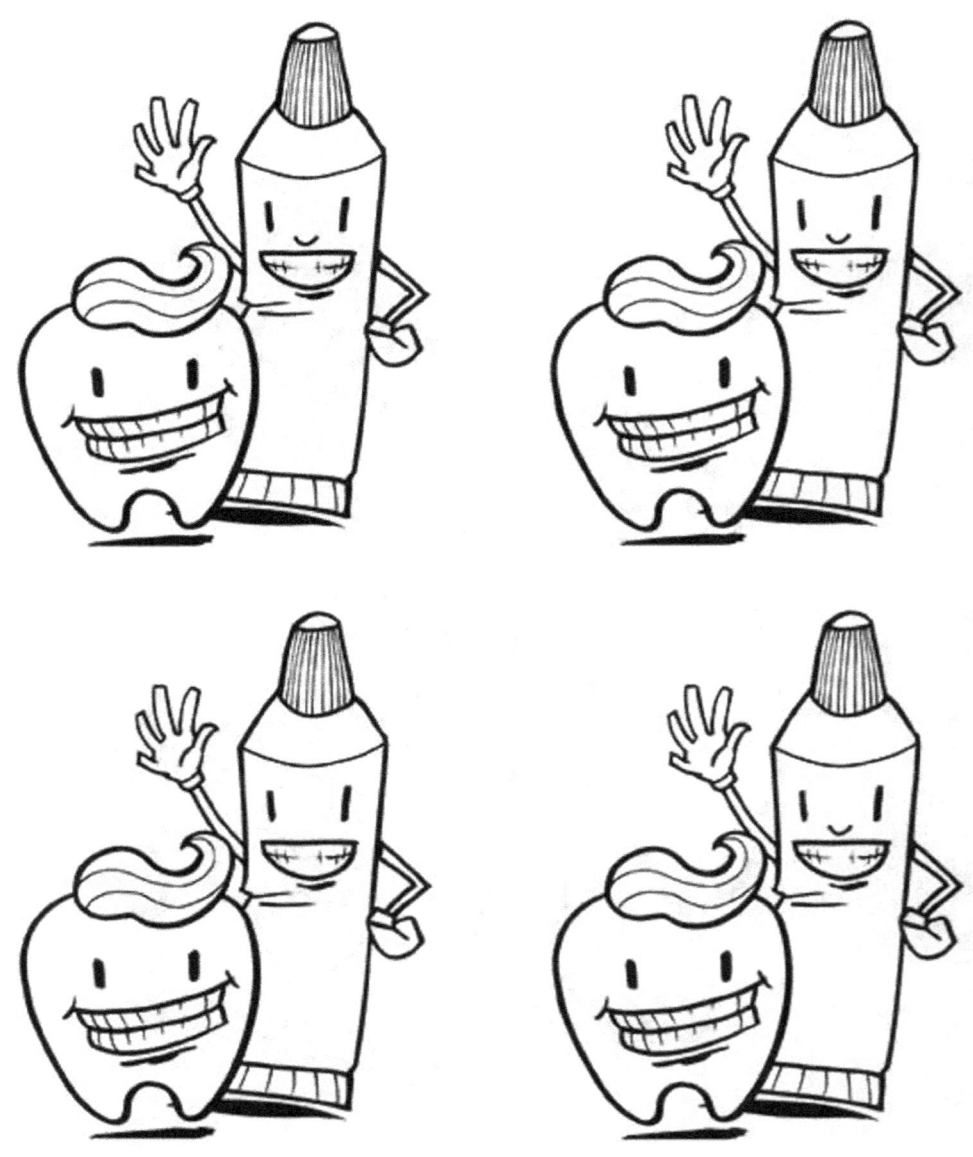

Picture Crossword

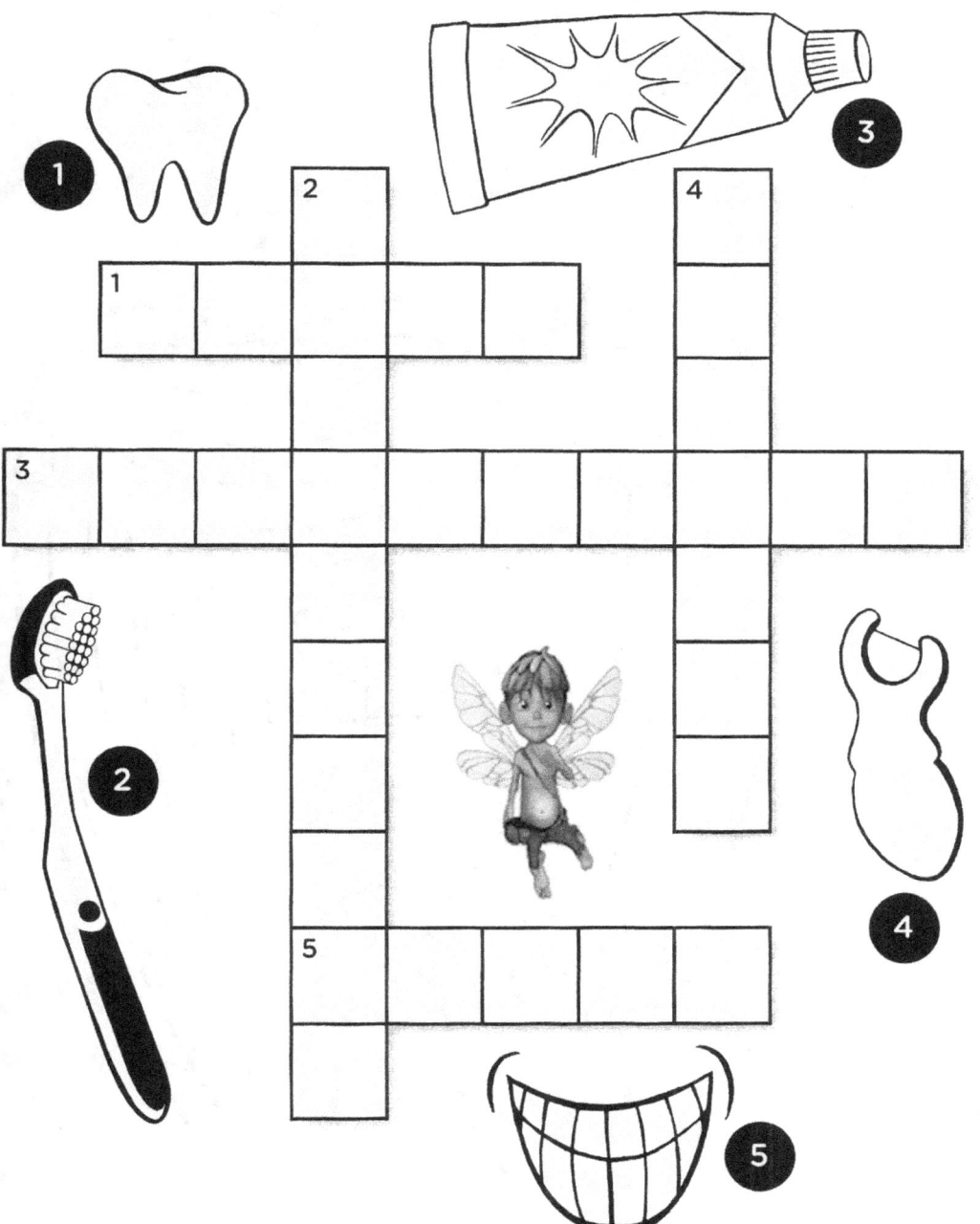

TOOTHY MAZE

OH NO! THERE IS A TOOTH BUG
HIDING IN THIS TOOTH!

HELP THESE YOUNG DENTISTS FIND THEIR
WAY TO THE CENTER OF THE TOOTH TO
BATTLE CAVITY CAUSING BACTERIA.

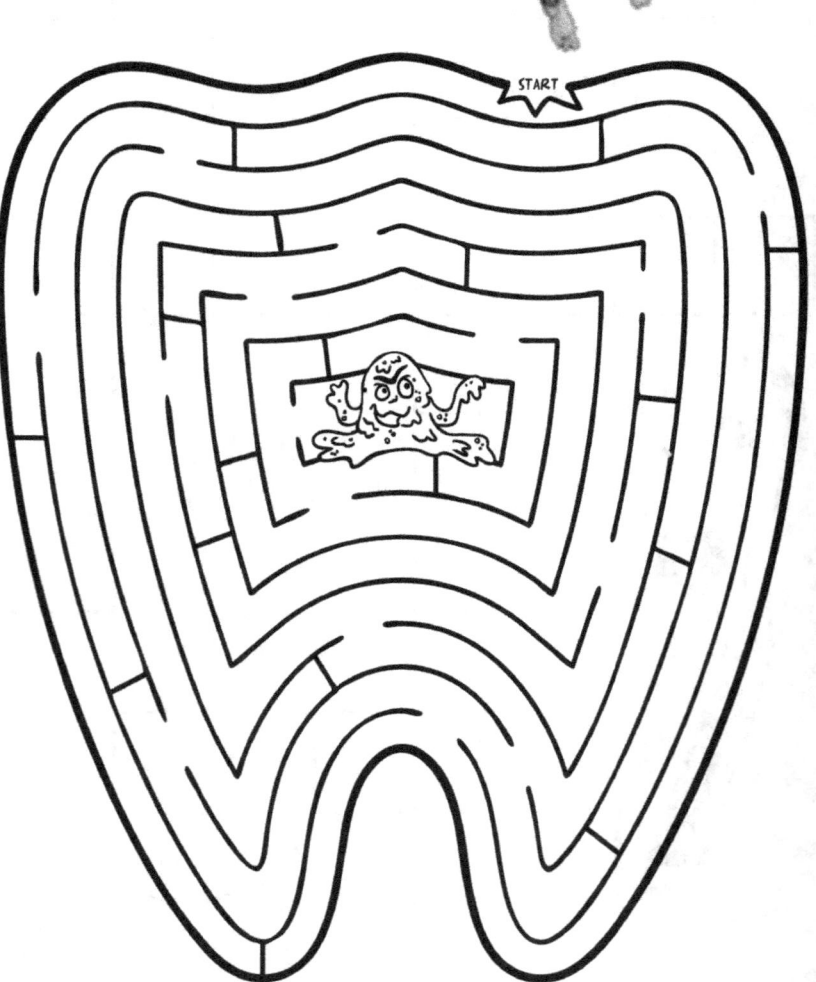

START

OKAY KIDS, IT'S TIME TO SHOW YOU THE
PROPER WAY TO BRUSH AND FLOSS YOUR
TEETH. SO GO GET YOUR TOOTHBRUSHES.

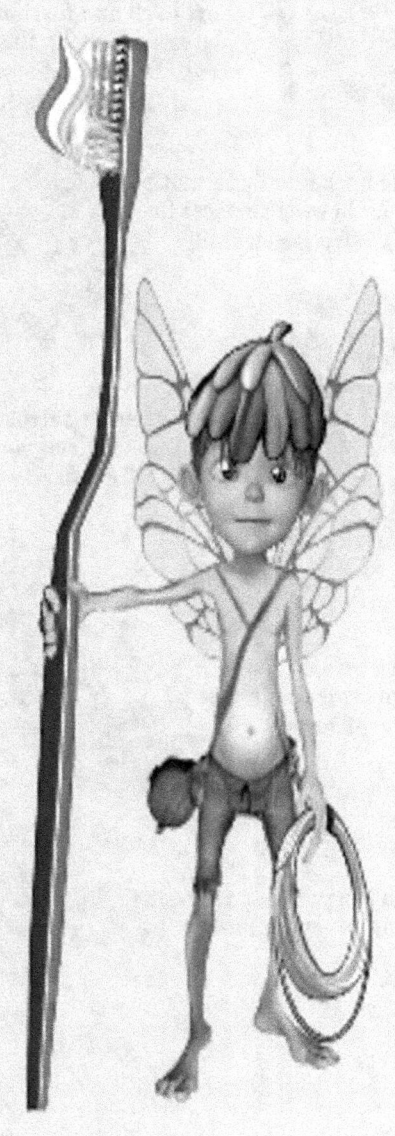

TOOTH BRUSH INSTRUCTIONS

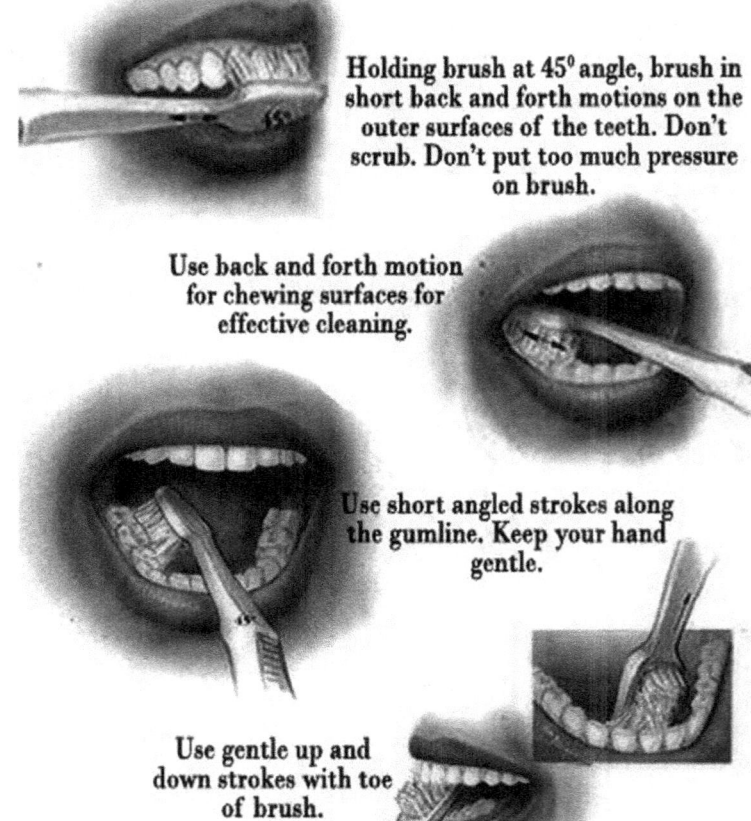

Holding brush at 45° angle, brush in short back and forth motions on the outer surfaces of the teeth. Don't scrub. Don't put too much pressure on brush.

Use back and forth motion for chewing surfaces for effective cleaning.

Use short angled strokes along the gumline. Keep your hand gentle.

Use gentle up and down strokes with toe of brush.

Brush tongue back to front using sweeping motion.

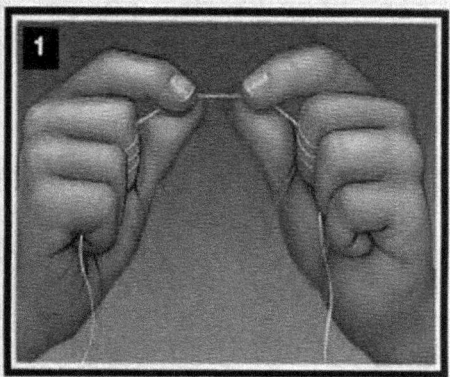

Wind 18" of floss around middle fingers of each hand. Pinch floss between thumbs and index fingers, leaving 1" - 2" length in between. Use thumbs to direct floss between upper teeth.

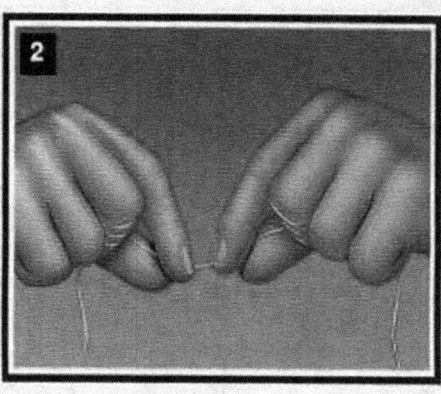

Keep a 1" - 2" length of floss taut between fingers. Use index fingers to guide floss between contacts of the lower teeth.

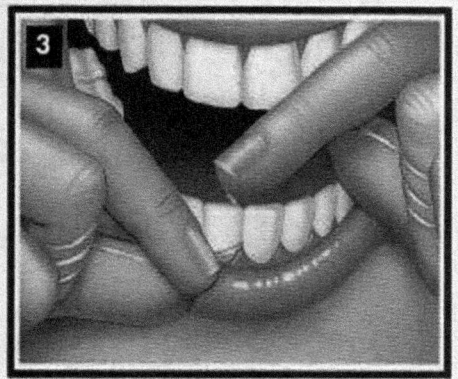

Gently guide floss between the teeth by using a zig-zag motion. DO NOT SNAP FLOSS BETWEEN YOUR TEETH. Contour floss around the side of the tooth.

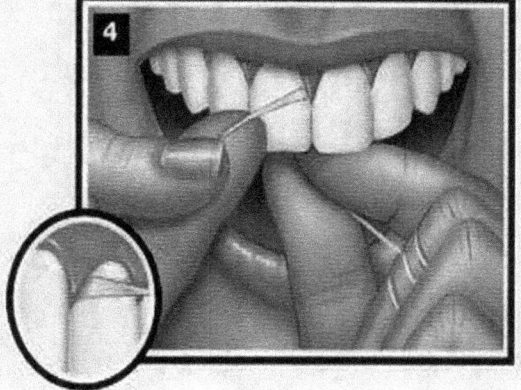

Slide floss up and down against the tooth surface and under the gumline. Floss each tooth thoroughly with a clean section of floss.

FLOSSING INSTRUCTIONS

THE END

FOR MORE INFORMATION PLEASE VISIT
www.plaquepixiebooks.com

www.ingramcontent.com/pod-product-compliance
Lightning Source LLC
Chambersburg PA
CBHW070945290526
45795CB00003B/1143